A Fun Guide for Kids to Keep Their Body & Space Clean

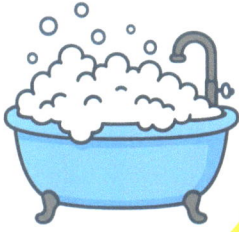

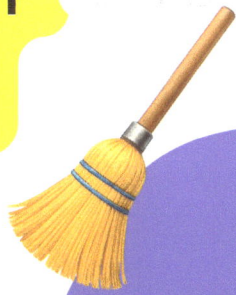

Why Being Clean Makes You Cool

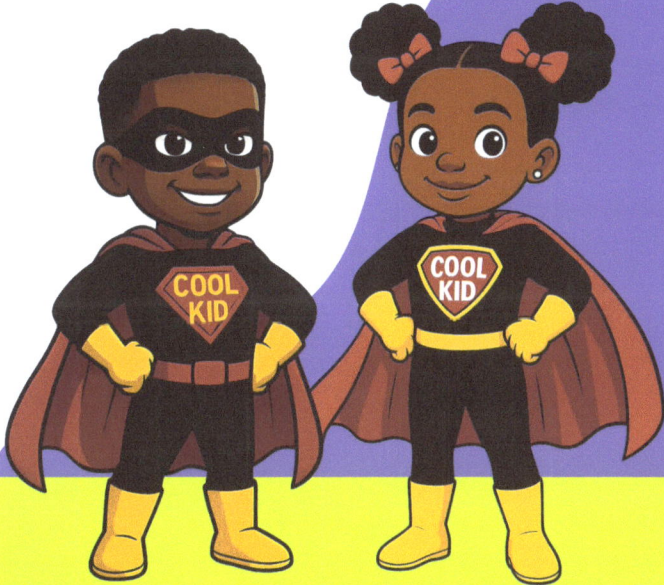

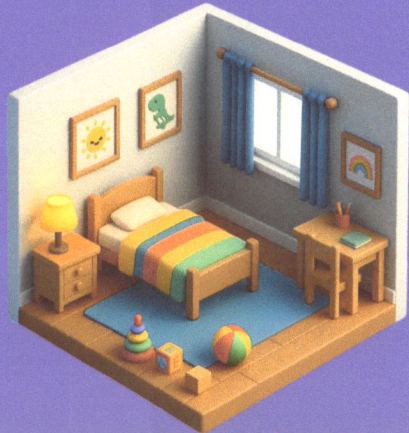

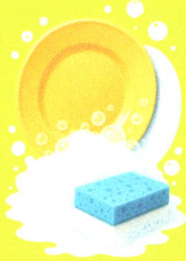

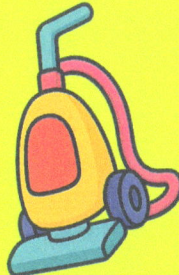

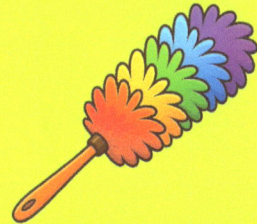

By: Jamila N. Houston

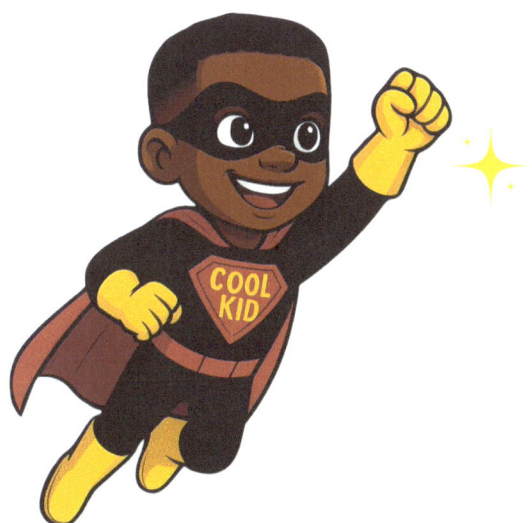

This book belongs to

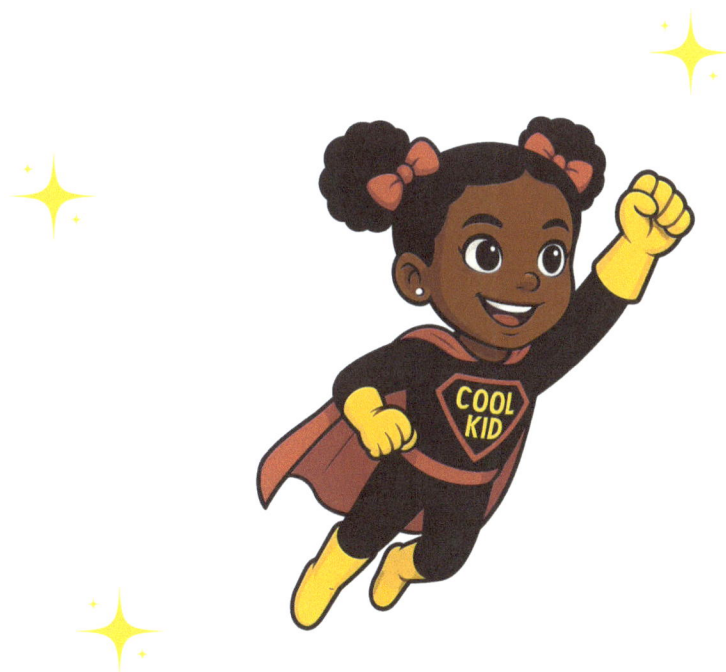

_____

"A Fun Guide for Kids to Keep Their Body & Space Clean: Why Being Clean Makes You Cool" is an engaging and empowering guide designed just for kids ages 6 to 12.

This fun, colorful, and interactive book helps young readers understand the importance of keeping both their body clean on the inside and outside—and how that connects to taking care of their home and personal space too!

Rooted in the uplifting message that "cleanliness is next to godliness", this guide uses playful language, checklists, games, and fun facts to make hygiene and cleaning feel exciting instead of a chore.

Your child will learn:
- How a clean body helps them feel confident, healthy, and energized.
- Why drinking water and eating healthy foods make them stronger and smarter.
- How tidying up their space leads to better sleep, focus, and happiness.
- Monthly and weekly cleaning habits that builds responsibility and independence.

Each section includes mini challenges, cool kid tips, and positive reinforcement to help children build lifelong habits in a way that feels fun, not forced.

Whether you're a parent, teacher, or caregiver, this guide is a perfect tool to help kids become more responsible, confident, and proud of themselves and their environment.

WELCOME COOL KID! Get ready to learn how to keep both your body and your space clean and happy! ✨

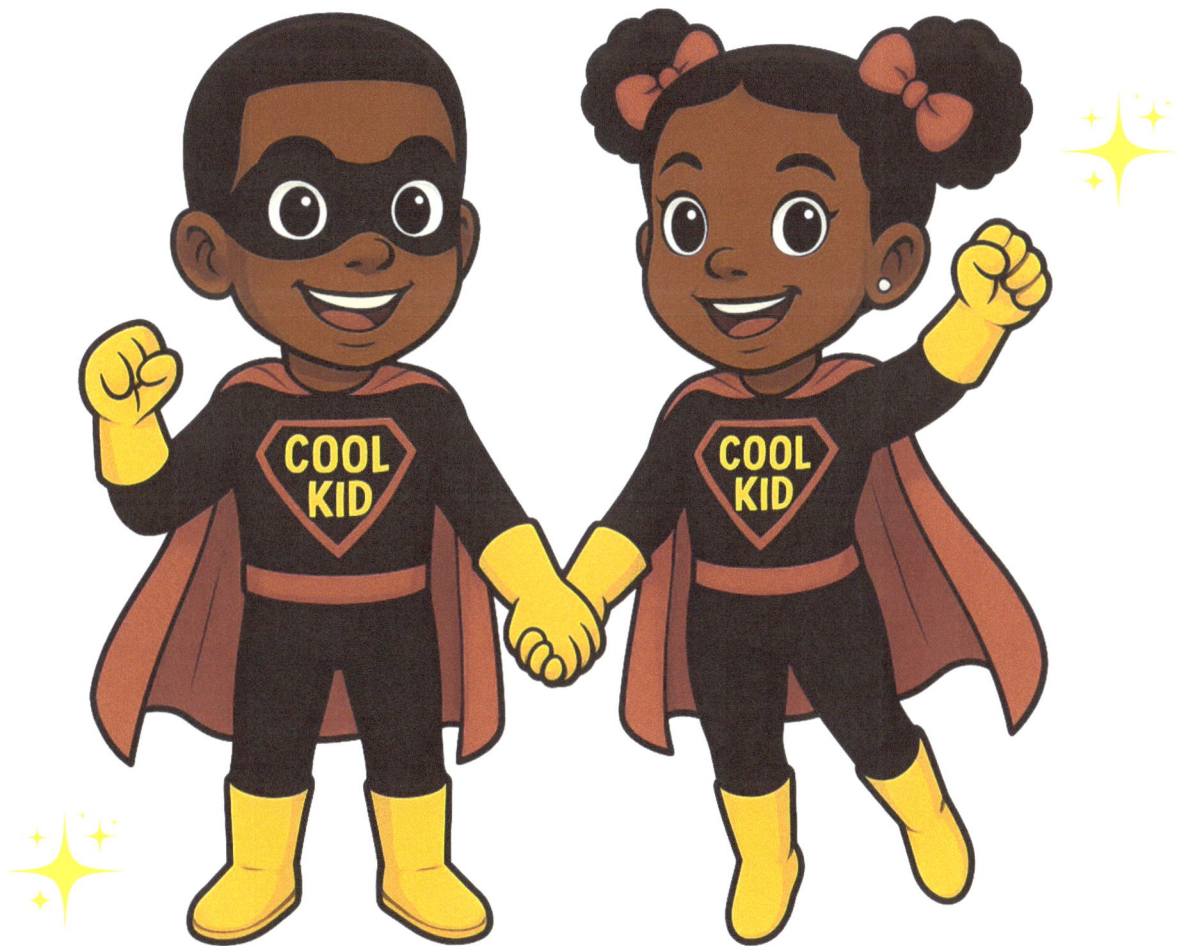

SECTION 1: MY BODY

1. Clean on the outside

Daily Hygiene Checklist:

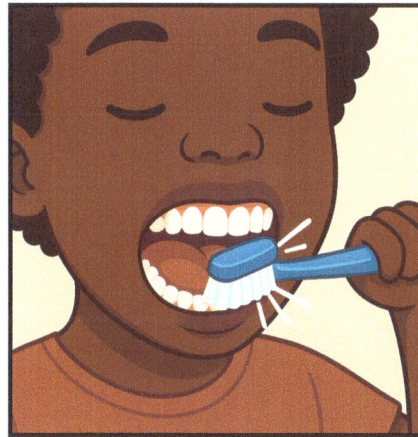

- Brushing your teeth

- Washing your face

- Taking a bath or shower

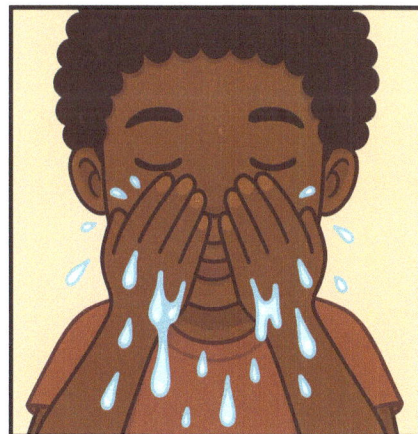

- Washing your hands

FUN FACT BOX:

Keeping your skin clean helps prevent getting sick. Your skin is the biggest organ.

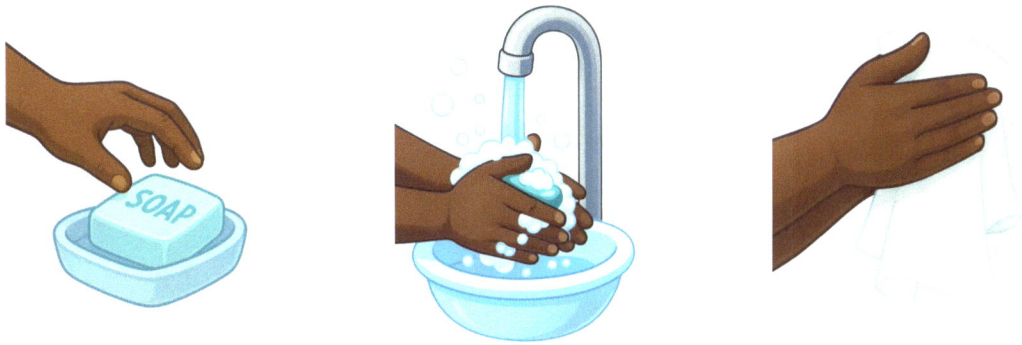

1. Wet Your Hands
- Turn on the tap and wet your hands with clean, warm water.

2. Add Soap
- Pump some soap onto your hands (one squirt is usually enough).

3. Rub Your Hands Together
- Rub them together to make bubbles! Make sure to scrub the palms, the back of your hands, between your fingers, and under your nails.

- Keep scrubbing for at least 20 seconds – try singing the "Happy Birthday" song twice.

4. Rinse Your Hands
- Put your hands back under the water and rinse off all the soap.

5. Dry Your Hands
- Use a clean towel to dry your hands or let them air dry.

6. Turn Off the Tap
- If possible, use the towel to turn off the tap, especially if you're in a public bathroom.

By following these steps, you can make sure their hands are squeaky clean and ready to keep germs away!

2. Clean on the inside

Healthy Eating Tips:

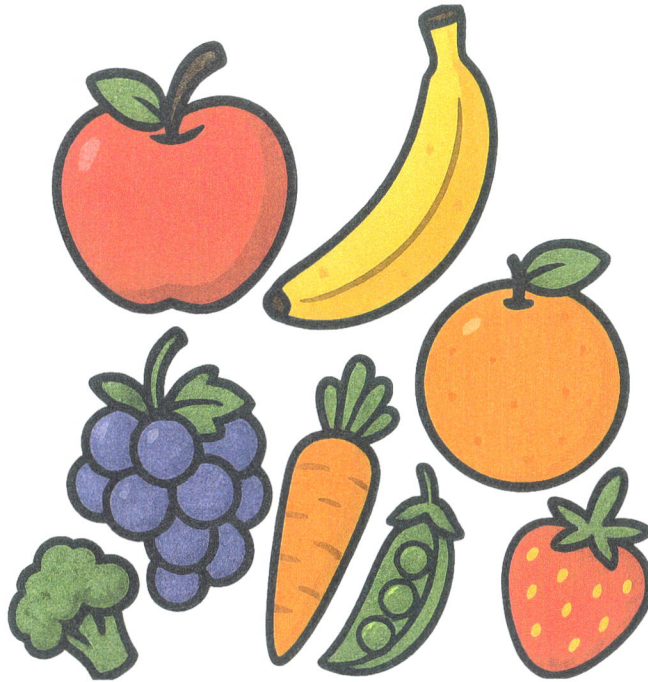

Eating good fruits and vegetables is like giving your body a bath from the inside!

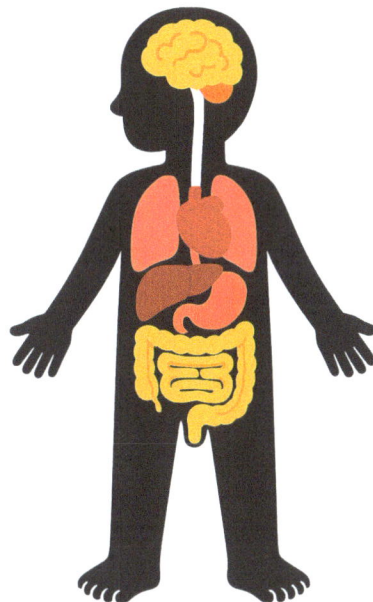

Daily Water Intake

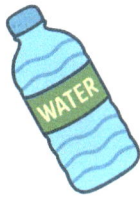
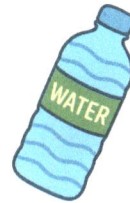

DAILY GOAL _____

SUNDAY
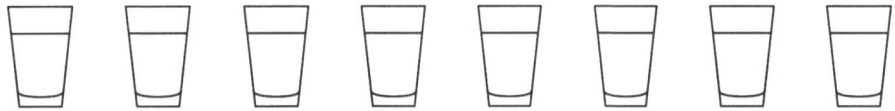

MONDAY
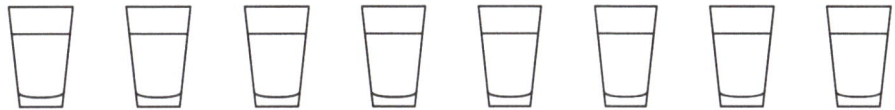

TUESDAY
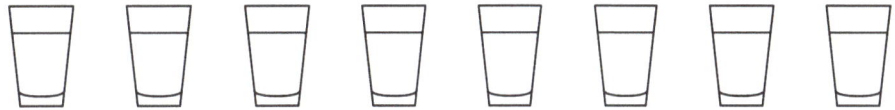

WEDNESDAY
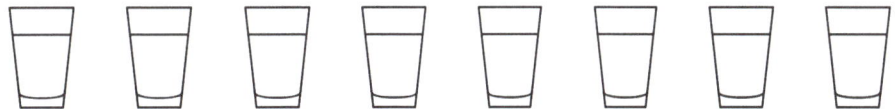

THURSDAY
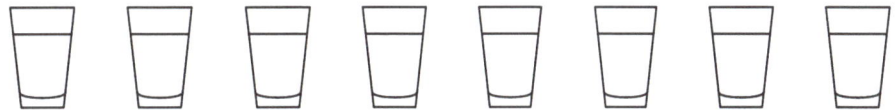

FRIDAY
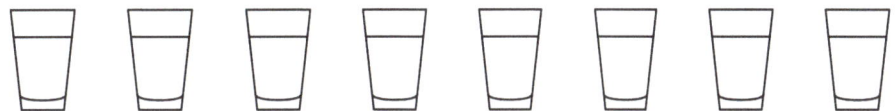

SATURDAY
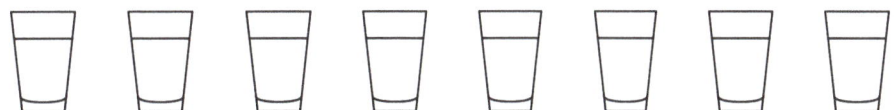

A fun way for kids to mark how many glasses of water they drink each day

Draw your favorite fruit, veggie, or healthy meal:

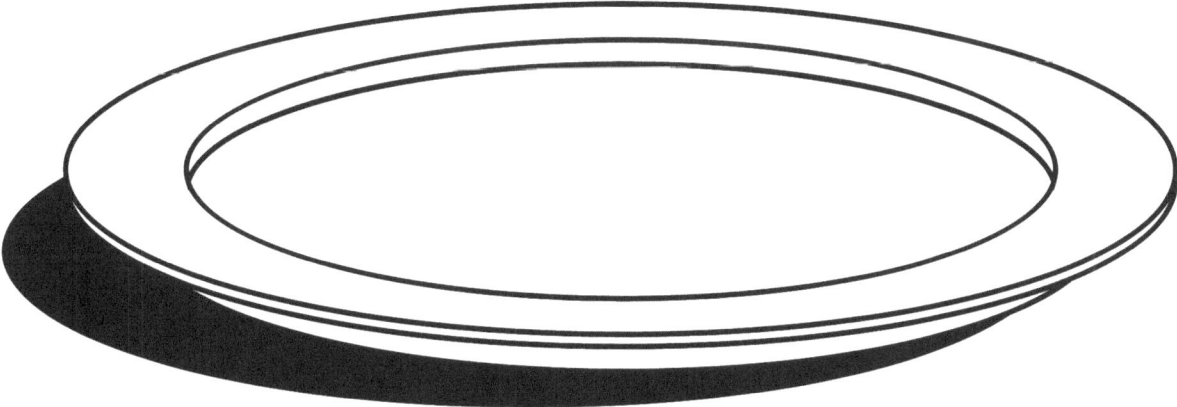

3. Body & Space Connection:

"Just like you need to clean your body to stay healthy, you need to clean the spaces where you live and play to feel good, too!"

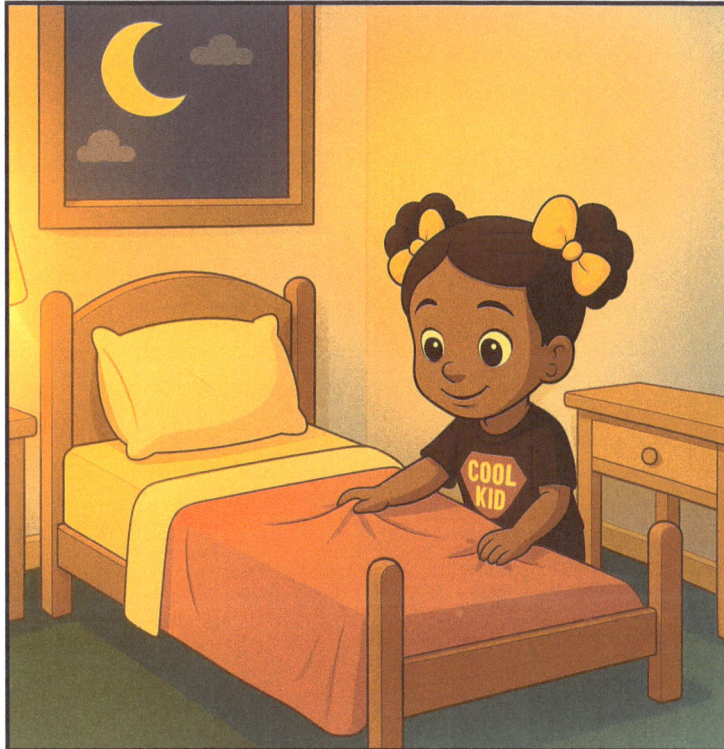

Fun Fact:
Keeping your room clean helps you sleep better at night!

Hygiene Cleaning Match Game

Directions:
Match the pictures of cleaning tools to the task. Draw lines to each item to match.

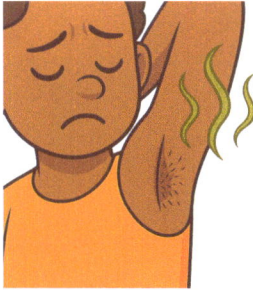

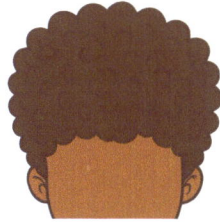

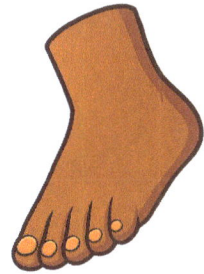

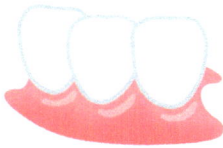

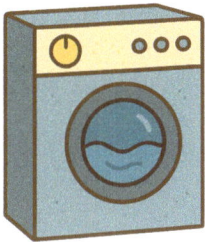

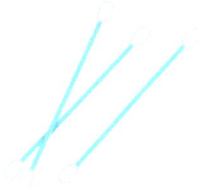

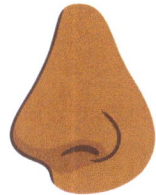

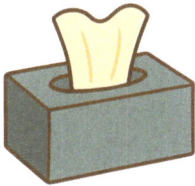

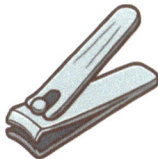

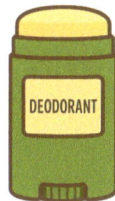

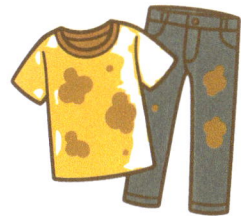

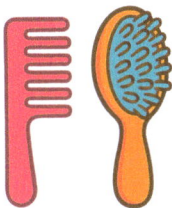

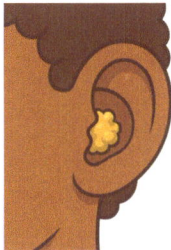

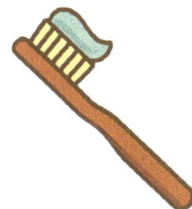

Fun Facts and Tips....clean is COOL!

COOL FACT:
Your skin protects your body like a superhero suit! It keeps germs out and helps you feel things like hot, cold, and soft textures.

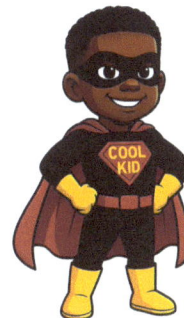

Why It's Cool:
Keeping your skin clean by washing it daily helps stop germs from making you sick.

COOL FACT:
Germs can hide on your hands and spread to everything you touch! Singing the ABC song while washing your hands for at least 20 seconds washes them away.

Why It's Cool:
Your mouth has over 700 types of bacteria some are good, some are bad!

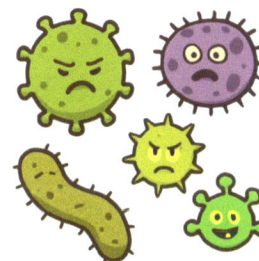

COOL FACT:
That's why brushing your teeth is super important. It removes the bad bacteria that can cause stinky breath and cavities. Also floss every night to get in between your teeth!

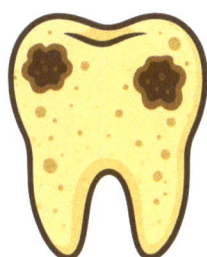

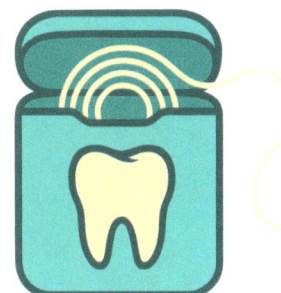

Fun Facts and Tips....clean is COOL!

COOL FACT:

Your body is mostly made of water! Water helps your muscles stay strong and your brain focused.

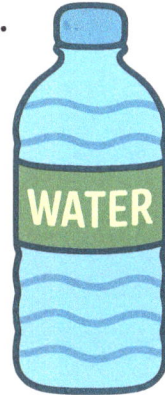

Why It's Cool:

When you drink enough water, you feel less tired and you'll have more energy to play.

COOL FACT:

Fruits, veggies, and water help your body run like a race car. Junk food can make you feel tired and slow.

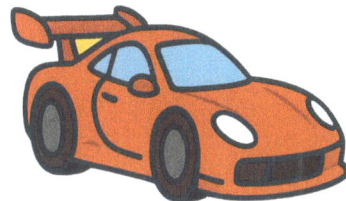

COOL KID CHALLENGE:

Try eating at least one fruit or veggie at every meal. What's your favorite? Write it below.

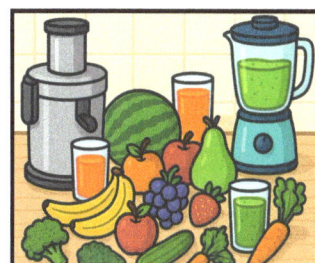

_____

_____

Let's play a Spelling Game! Unscramble the letters for fruits and veggies, fill in the blanks. Spell the words correctly.

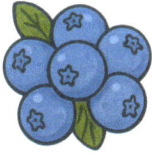

E B L U R R I E S B E

_ _ _ _ _ _ _ _ _ _

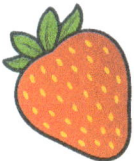

T S R W A E B R R Y

_ _ _ _ _ _ _ _ _ _

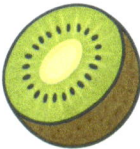

W I K I

_ _ _ _

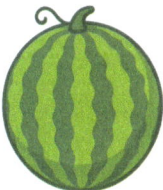

T E R W A N E L O M

_ _ _ _ _ _ _ _ _ _

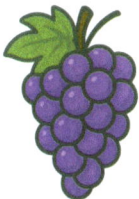

S R G A P E

_ _ _ _ _ _

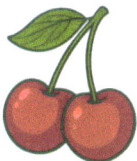

H E C R I E R S

_ _ _ _ _ _ _

MONTHLY CLEANING CHECKLIST

◯ **Change your sheets and pillowcases**

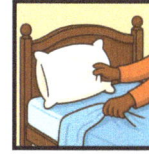

◯ **Dust off the back of your headboard**

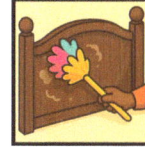

◯ **Wash your blankets & stuffed animals**

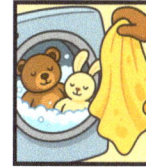

◯ **Sweep or Vacuum under your bed**

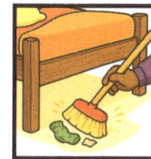

◯ **Wipe down light switches**

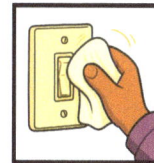

◯ **Wipe down doorknobs**

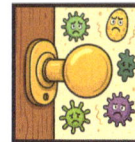

◯ **Throw out old toothbrushes (replace every 3 months)**

◯ **Wipe down tablets**

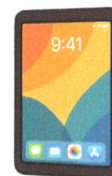

◯ **Organize your book bag**

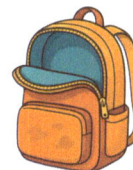

◯ **Wipe down controllers**

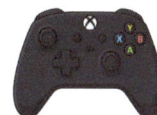

Cut this out and put it up on your wall.

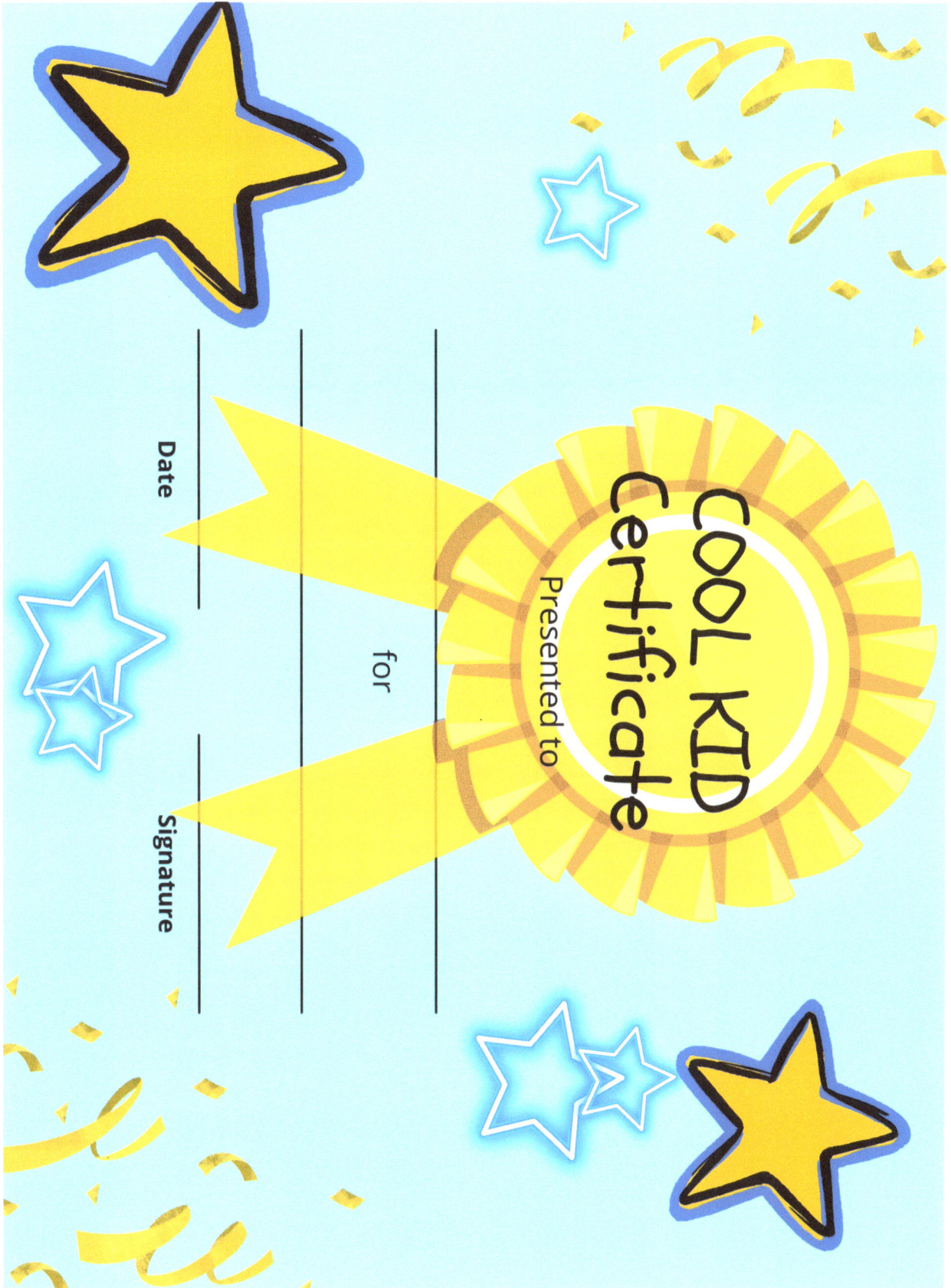

COOL KID Certificate

Presented to

Date

for

Signature

COOL KID AFFIRMATIONS

l. I take care of my space, and it takes care of me.

2. A healthy body gives me energy to play and learn.

3. Cleaning my space makes me feel happy and calm.

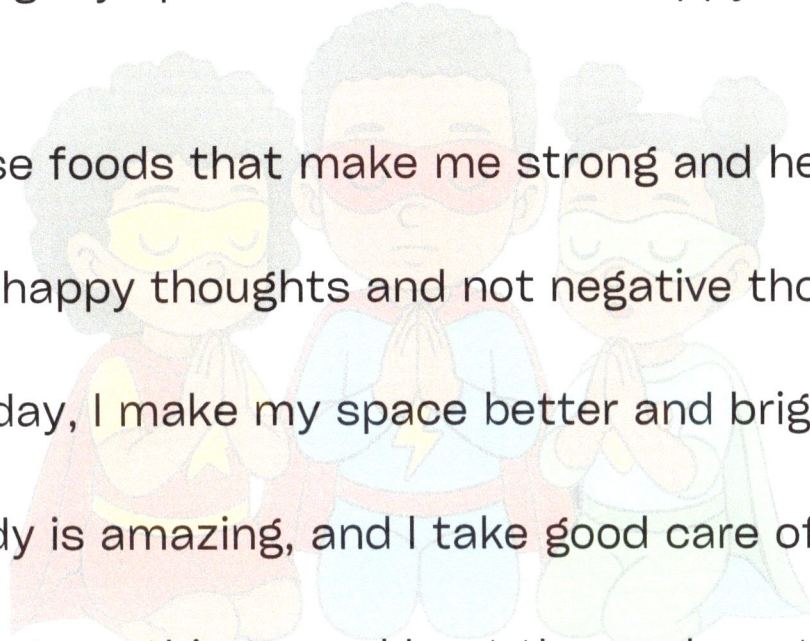

4. I choose foods that make me strong and healthy.

5. I think happy thoughts and not negative thoughts.

6. Every day, I make my space better and brighter.

7. My body is amazing, and I take good care of it.

8. I respect my things, and I put them where they belong.

9. Drinking water keeps my body happy and healthy.

10. I am grateful for my home, my health, and my happiness.

Cool Kid Crossword Puzzle

H	K	T	E	N	E	R	G	Y	N	A	L	B	F	U
R	M	I	N	D	K	G	R	A	T	E	F	U	L	U
E	T	L	I	M	C	I	K	L	H	H	O	H	I	C
S	S	E	V	B	L	X	J	O	E	V	D	F	O	G
T	T	N	F	R	E	P	P	V	A	H	Y	R	K	Z
K	R	A	Q	H	A	W	E	E	L	Q	H	I	S	B
K	O	J	G	E	N	M	A	L	T	F	O	C	U	S
R	N	U	R	A	E	K	C	R	H	Z	K	Y	V	Y
D	G	U	A	R	T	G	E	N	Y	B	C	D	B	N
B	J	O	Y	T	W	U	C	I	N	O	M	W	R	H
S	P	I	R	I	T	Y	R	W	O	D	C	A	A	S
M	I	S	S	A	F	R	U	N	L	Y	A	T	V	T
Q	Z	S	A	J	C	S	M	I	L	E	L	E	E	N
N	B	E	K	I	N	D	N	Y	T	I	M	R	A	H
D	C	X	Y	T	A	C	H	I	L	D	R	E	N	S

SMILE   HEART   CALM   CHILDREN

BODY   LOVE   STRONG   GRATEFUL   BRAVE

SPIRIT   MIND   CLEAN   WATER   ENERGY

PEACE   REST   JOY   KIND   HEALTHY   FOCUS

NOTES

✦ NOTES ✦

_____

_____

_____

_____

_____

_____

_____

_____

_____

_____

_____

NOTES

✨ NOTES ✨

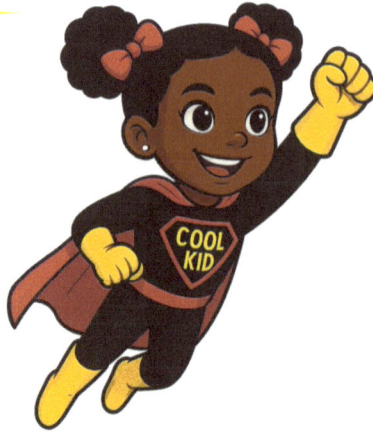

THANK YOU

For

BEING A COOL KID!

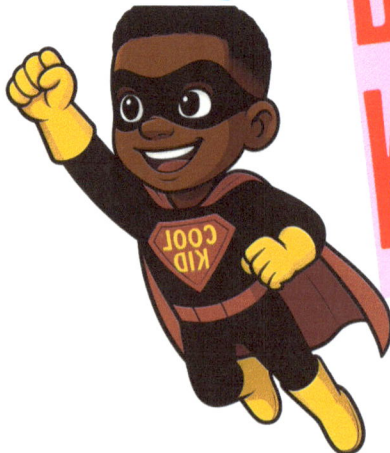

www.ingramcontent.com/pod-product-compliance
Lightning Source LLC
Chambersburg PA
CBHW060825270326
41931CB00002B/64